Chair Yoga for Weight Loss

Alex Harper

"For the wise and resilient elders who inspire us with your strength and wisdom, this book is dedicated to your enduring vitality. May it enrich your journey toward wellness and joy."

Alex Harper

VIDEO BONUS

To get your **FREE** lifetime 🎥**VIDEO ACCESS**🎥 to our invigorating **CHAIR YOGA EXERCISES** just scan the QR code above or enter this link https://bit.ly/CYWL-video into your search browser.

Want also **FREE BOOKS** for the rest of your LIFE?

Join our VIP club now by scanning the QR code to get **FREE** access to all our future books.

We ONLY send you an email when we launch a NEW BOOK. NO SPAM. Never. Ever!

Just an email with **YOUR FREE BOOK**.

Get ready to elevate your fitness journey!

TABLE OF CONTENTS

BEFORE YOU BEGIN

Thank you for picking up this book! I've dedicated myself to ensuring it's filled with accurate and safe guidance. Every detail has been thoroughly fact-checked and cited to offer trustworthy advice. This book is here to support your weight loss journey through Chair Yoga, whether you're just starting out or looking to deepen your practice.

I'd be grateful if you could leave a review after reading. Your feedback helps me continue creating content that benefits others on their wellness path. Wishing you success and enjoyment on this transformative journey!

INTRODUCTION

Have you ever wondered why you feel fatigued and lack the energy to move from one place to another? Well, you've found the right book to help address those challenges. Thanks to the latest scientific breakthroughs, we now have a clearer understanding of how exercise and yoga can positively impact our lives. In particular, we recognize how essential they are for maintaining energy, mobility, and overall well-being as we age.

For those with chronic conditions, regular exercise and yoga are crucial for maintaining muscle elasticity and enabling the performance of daily tasks with greater ease. When paired with proper sleep, meditation, and balanced routines, these practices can help elevate serotonin levels (the "happy hormone"), making life more joyful and rewarding.

I'm Alex Harper, a certified fitness expert who has guided hundreds of individuals toward achieving their fitness goals. As we age, it's vital to maintain strong, flexible muscles, and that's exactly why I've packed over a decade of experience into this book, specifically tailored to meet the needs of seniors.

Fitness doesn't have an age limit. No matter your age, staying fit is within your reach. The key is finding the motivation to stay consistent on your journey. I understand the unique challenges seniors face when it comes to fitness, and my experience has helped countless clients achieve not only their health goals but also a renewed sense of confidence and joy in their daily lives. I've had the privilege of helping thousands of people transform their fitness and well-being, and I'm excited to share this knowledge with you.

Chair yoga is a unique practice that can be enjoyed by fitness enthusiasts of all ages, not just those who find traditional yoga on the mat difficult. Even if you simply prefer not to practice yoga on the floor, chair yoga provides a comfortable and accessible alternative to pursue your fitness goals.

In this book, I'll also introduce you to the principles of weight loss through chair yoga. By combining mindful movements, breathing exercises, and a sustainable approach to wellness, you can lose weight in a way that respects your body's capabilities and promotes lasting results. So get ready for a journey that takes you deep into both your physical and mental well-being, helping you achieve a healthier, more energized version of yourself!

CHAPTER 1:
UNLOCKING THE POWER OF CHAIR YOGA

"Yoga is not about touching your toes,
it's about what you learn on the way down."

–Jigar Gor

Chair yoga is a form of yoga that helps you slide into your daily exercise and meditation regimen with considerable ease. Granted, most of us tend to rethink our dedication to getting lean and having a tranquil state of mind when we realize we need to do tons of preparatory work. However, using a chair that can be placed anywhere in your home to do yoga exercises has changed how people approach yoga.

Indubitably, yoga has become more accessible. Chair yoga helps build strength, resilience, and coordination in seniors, who may struggle to achieve the same through traditional yoga. Seniors find it very easy to do yoga on a chair, as it helps with their mobility. They can ease into their chair yoga regimen gradually.

The Benefits of Chair Yoga

The major benefit of chair yoga is that it helps keep the parts of your body that you're not meant to move in position so you can focus on the other parts of your body that you're meant to move. Seniors mostly suffer from chronic medical conditions and mobility issues stemming from arthritis. This calls for an exercise routine that is relatively easy to adopt for seniors. Doing these exercises in a sitting position in a comfy chair makes it easy for the elderly to focus on the correct movement of the limbs. The following are some benefits of chair yoga:

- Augmented strength and flexibility
- Improved balance
- Better cardiovascular health
- Reduced tendency to fall and improved mood

Improved Mobility, Strength, and Flexibility

Practicing a pose daily strengthens your body and makes your muscles flexible. The muscle fibers show better tensile strength, allowing you to perform tasks more efficiently, without feeling pain or fatigue.

Improved Balance and Reduced Tendency to Fall

The ability to balance yourself diminishes with age, but yoga can make you more aware of your limits. It helps you hone your senses and balance your body. As pain and discomfort start to dampen, your balance and agility improve.

Better Cardiovascular Health and Posture

Daily physical activity makes the heart more efficient at pumping blood all around the body and fortifies the muscles, which improves posture. Furthermore, the tendons holding the muscles and bones together become stronger as do the ligaments. As such, the muscles can lift heavier weights and perform more tasks. Seniors can become more agile, especially when they become more invested in their daily activities and hobbies, such as gardening and wildcrafting.

Principles of Chair Yoga

Principles help us understand what we are doing and why we are doing it. Without principles, repeated actions can easily become meaningless, and we will become unmotivated and bored. Chair Yoga has a set of principles that it operates on, and understanding them will help you reap the most benefits out of your practice. The core principles in Yoga are alignment, stability, and breathwork.

Alignment and Stability

According to the Bone Health and Osteoporosis Foundation (n.d.), alignment refers to how the spine, head, shoulders, pelvis, hips, knees, and ankles line up with each other. Improper alignment and form can lead to uncomfortable conditions like slipped discs in the lower back. Below are some simple alignment steps that you can practice while performing Chair Yoga to ensure that you avoid injuries and enhance your workout.

Neutral Spine

Your back has three curves: one in the neck, one in the thoracic region (middle back), and one in the lower back. Maintaining a neutral spine means that all three of those regions are aligned. To find this alignment, lie down on your back, then bend your knees with your feet flat on the mat.

Rest your body on the mat, ensuring that you have no tension or tightness in any area, then tuck your pelvis by drawing your navel toward your spine. There should be little space between the mat and your back; if there isn't, tilt the pelvic region upwards away from the floor.

Shoulder Position

Maintain good shoulder alignment by pulling your scapulae (shoulder blades) downward. Release any tension in your shoulders by inhaling as you lift them, then exhaling as you gently lower them back down.

Head Alignment

Pay extra attention to your head alignment during Chair Yoga because we normally tend to keep it shrugged, bent, or however we feel like. To make sure your head is aligned with your spine, shoulders, and pelvis, imagine an invisible line is tied to the center of your head and is pulling your head upward.

Allow this invisible line to pull your head until your neck is extended and no longer curved. This shouldn't make you feel uncomfortable, but if it does, slowly drop your eyes down to the floor and let your head follow until you no longer feel any discomfort or tension.

Pelvic Alignment

Tuck your tailbone inward and engage your lower abdominal muscles to stabilize your pelvis. To make sure that your pelvis is in alignment with your spine, stand with your back against a wall. Next, put your hand in the space that your back makes with the wall. Then, tuck your pelvis in, lift your chest, and engage your shoulder blades—all while making sure your rib cage is expanded.

Once you've done so, check if the space between your lower back and the wall is minimal to none. That will also depend on the level of your strength and flexibility, so don't fret if you find that there is still a lot of space when you do that. As you continue practicing Chair Yoga, you will get more flexible.

Hip and Knee Alignment

Your hips also have to remain in alignment with your knees. Align them by maintaining a parallel position between your hips and knees. You can also test your alignment by standing hip-width apart and avoiding bending your knees or locking them in too tightly. Don't let your knees collapse inward or push them too far outward.

Strengthening Core Stability

A strong core will help you enhance stability when practicing Chair Yoga. It will also help improve your posture and balance. If you find it difficult to maintain body alignment and stability, focus on building strength in your core muscles.

The stronger your core, the more precise your movements will be; and for us who want a better midsection, a strong core will give you those washboard abs!

CHAPTER 2:

PRINCIPLES OF WEIGHT LOSS

Getting older doesn't mean giving up on staying fit. Sure, our bodies change, but that just means we must change how we think about weight loss. In this chapter, we're going to discuss what really matters when it comes to shedding a few pounds as we age. Rather than talk about crash diets or spending hours at the gym, we'll look at how our bodies work differently now and what that means for keeping healthy. From what we eat to how we move, we'll cover the basics that make a real difference.

Healthy Eating Habits for Weight Loss

We all know that food choices play a big role in managing weight. Our bodies don't burn calories as quickly as they used to, so we need to be a little more careful about what and when we eat. Below are some key tips to help with this process.

Eating Less in the Evening

As the day winds down, our bodies require less energy to function, which means the food we consume in the evening is more likely to be stored as fat than to be used as immediate fuel. This effect becomes even more pronounced as we age because our bodies become less efficient at burning calories.

To prevent this, try to keep evening meals smaller and lighter. Focus on nutrient-dense but lower-calorie options that satisfy your hunger without overloading your system. Great choices include soups, salads, and lean proteins such as chicken or fish.

Moreover, eating your last meal three hours before you sleep gives your body enough time to digest the food you've eaten (Kinsey & Ormsbee, 2015).

Increasing Vegetable Intake for Satiety

Vegetables are essential for weight loss because they are rich in fiber, which is a nutrient that supports digestion and keeps you full longer even when you're eating fewer calories. What's more, vegetables are packed with vitamins, minerals, and other healthy nutrients that are good for your body.

There are several fun and tasty ways to sneak more veggies into your meals. For instance, you can blend leafy greens such as spinach or kale into smoothies for a nutritious boost without compromising on flavor. Another idea is to bulk up soups and stews by adding carrots, celery, or tomatoes.

Eating More Protein

People who eat a high-protein breakfast feel fuller and eat fewer calories throughout the day than those who skip breakfast or eat a low-protein meal (Leidy et al., 2013). This happens largely due to the *thermic effect of food*, which refers to the energy required for the digestion, absorption, and metabolism of nutrients. Protein has a much higher thermic effect than fats or carbohydrates, meaning the body expends more energy digesting protein-rich foods.

In fact, digesting protein burns approximately *20–30% of the calories* present in it, while digesting fats and carbohydrates burns only 0–3% and 5–10% of the calories present in them, respectively. Protein is not only essential for muscle preservation but is also an effective tool for weight management, as it helps boost metabolism and reduce overall calorie intake by increasing satiety (Westerterp, 2004).

Furthermore, protein is super important for keeping your muscles strong and healthy. This matters because muscles are little calorie-burning machines in your body. As such, more muscles mean more calories burned even while just sitting!

Excellent protein sources include eggs, lean meats such as chicken or fish, and plant-based options such as tofu and legumes. Seniors who may have difficulty chewing tougher meats can opt for soft proteins such as scrambled eggs or Greek yogurt, which are easy to digest but still provide plenty of protein.

Making Smarter Food Choices

- **Low Glycemic Index (GI) Carbs**: Not all carbs are the same. Some are like speed demons, rushing into your bloodstream and causing all sorts of chaos. Others are like slow, steady tortoises, giving you energy without the drama. These slower carbs are what we call *low GI carbs*. Great examples of low-GI carbs include *brown rice, basmati rice, whole grains, and oats*. But why does this matter? A spike in your blood sugar levels results in your body releasing a hormone called insulin to deal with all that sugar. If this happens too often, your body might start ignoring insulin. This is called insulin resistance, and it can lead to weight gain and other health issues (Ludwig, 2002).

- **Sourdough vs. Regular Bread**: When it comes to bread, sourdough is often a healthier option compared to regular white or wheat bread. Well, it's all about the process. Sourdough bread is made using a fermentation process that creates beneficial bacteria. These little guys work hard to break down some of the carbs in the bread before it even reaches your plate. The result? A bread that's easier on your blood sugar levels (Scazzina et al., 2009). The fermentation process also makes the nutrients in the bread more easily available for your body to use. It's like the sourdough is doing some of the digestive work for you!

- **Healthy Potato Options**: Potatoes aren't bad if prepared properly—boiled, baked, or roasted without heavy fats. They're rich in *vitamins, potassium, and fiber*, especially with the skin on. Cooking methods also affect their GI. For example, potatoes that have been boiled and then cooled have a lower GI than baked ones (Fernandes et al., 2005). So, to keep potatoes healthy, focus on how they're prepared. Consider healthy options such as potato salads with boiled cooled potatoes or roasted wedges with olive oil and herbs.

- **Honey vs. Table Sugar**: When you need to sweeten your food, consider replacing table (refined) sugar with honey. Unlike table sugar, honey is a natural sweetener with added nutrients such as antioxidants, vitamins, and minerals (Bogdanov et al., 2008). Some studies have found that honey might have a gentler effect on your blood sugar than table sugar. People have a lower blood sugar response when they eat honey than when they eat the same amount of sugar (Abdulrhman et al., 2013).

- **Low-Fat Dairy Options**: Low-fat dairy products, such as *skim or 1% milk, low-fat yogurt, and reduced-fat cheeses*, offer the same essential nutrients as their full-fat counterparts, including calcium, protein, and vitamin D, without the added calories and saturated fat. But it's not just about weight loss. Low-fat dairy still gives you all the calcium you need for strong bones and teeth. It's also a great source of protein, which we know is important to feel full and maintain muscle mass. Some low-fat dairy products, such as yogurt, even come with probiotics, which are friendly bacteria that keep your gut happy (Fernández et al., 2017).

The Role of Movement in Weight Loss

Weight loss isn't just about what we eat; how we move matters too. For seniors, this doesn't mean grueling gym sessions. Instead, it's about incorporating movement into everyday life. Whether it's moving after meals to help with digestion or starting the day with gentle activity, every bit of movement counts.

Movement Throughout the Day

You might think that only intense exercises such as jogging or lifting weights can aid weight loss, but small, everyday movements can also help burn calories. Yep, you heard that right—you don't need the membership of a fancy gym or any expensive equipment to stay active. Tasks such as sweeping, vacuuming, cooking, walking to the mailbox, or folding laundry keep you moving and prevent long periods of sitting—benefiting your health and weight management.

Moving After Meals to Improve Insulin Sensitivity

After you eat, your body uses *insulin* to help transport sugar from the food you eat to your cells, where it's used for energy. This is called *insulin sensitivity,* which is essentially how well your body responds to insulin. When you improve your insulin sensitivity, your body can process sugar more effectively, which helps prevent excess fat storage.

A simple way to improve insulin sensitivity is by moving after meals. Doing something as easy as taking a short walk after eating can lower the fat concentration in your blood by up to 18% compared to just sitting down after a meal (Hijikata & Yamada, 2011). This means that even light movements after meals help your body burn sugar for energy instead of storing it as fat.

Pre-Breakfast Movement and Fasting

When you wake up in the morning, your body is in a special state. You haven't eaten for several hours, so your body is running low on the quick energy it gets from food. Scientists call this being in a "fasted state." When you're in this state, your body is more likely to burn fat for energy instead of the sugar from your last meal (Gonzalez et al., 2013).

So, if you can get your body moving before you eat breakfast, you're giving it a golden opportunity to burn some of that stored fat.

Moreover, pre-breakfast movement also helps improve your overall well-being. Starting the day with light exercise can increase energy, improve mood, and set a positive tone for the rest of the day.

Barriers to Burning Fat

Here, we'll break down some common barriers to burning fat and provide simple, actionable tips on overcoming them.

Inflammation and Weight Loss

Chronic inflammation can make it harder to shed those extra pounds. Inflammation is your body's natural response to injury or illness. However, when it sticks around for too long (chronic inflammation), it can affect your body's ability to burn fat, which, in turn, messes with your metabolism and makes it difficult for your cells to respond to insulin properly.

Solution: Include anti-inflammatory foods, such as fatty fish, nuts, and leafy greens, in your diet.

Glycemic Variability

Fluctuating blood sugar, also known as glycemic variability, can sabotage your weight loss goals. When your blood sugar spikes and crashes, you're more likely to feel hungry and tired and reach for unhealthy snacks. This leads to overindulgence, especially in high-sugar foods that are then stored as fat.

Solution: Stick to low-GI foods to keep your blood sugar stable and limit sugary snacks and drinks.

Cortisol and Stress

When you're stressed, your body releases a hormone called **cortisol**. High cortisol levels can lead to weight gain, especially around the belly. Stress can make your body store more fat and slow down your metabolism. Moreover, when you're stressed, you might be more likely to eat comfort foods high in sugar or fat.

Solution: Manage stress with techniques such as yoga, meditation, and deep breathing. We'll go into more detail about these techniques in later chapters.

Sleep Deprivation

Did you know that not getting enough sleep can make you hungrier? A lack of sleep affects two important hormones: *ghrelin and leptin.* Ghrelin tells you when you're hungry and leptin tells you when you're full. When you're sleep-deprived, ghrelin levels go up and leptin levels go down, meaning you're more likely to overeat. Poor sleep also slows down your metabolism, making it harder to burn fat.

Solution: Get enough rest to support weight loss by regulating hunger hormones and metabolism.

Frequent Non-Controlled Snacking

If you find yourself snacking throughout the day, it's easy to lose track of how much you're eating. *Mindless snacking* can be a major roadblock to weight loss because those extra calories add up quickly.

Solution: Practice mindful eating by eating balanced meals, staying hydrated, and choosing protein-rich snacks such as yogurt, nuts, or cheese.

Not Moving Enough or Overdoing Exercise

Exercise is a non-negotiable part of any weight loss plan, but too little movement slows down your metabolism, whereas overdoing it can lead to fatigue and injury.

This is especially important for older adults because they are more prone to joint problems and slow recovery times.

Solution: Find a balanced exercise routine that keeps you active without overexertion.

Hormonal Imbalances and Weight Loss

Aging causes hormone changes, which can affect how easily we lose weight. Hormonal imbalances can slow down metabolism and make it harder to burn fat. For example, a decrease in estrogen levels in women during menopause can lead to weight gain.

Solution: Eat more cruciferous vegetables such as broccoli to help balance hormones and reduce exposure to chemicals such as BPA by using glass or stainless-steel containers.

Micronutrient Deficiencies

Sometimes, weight loss is stalled because your body lacks important vitamins and minerals. Micronutrient deficiencies, such as those in vitamin D, magnesium, or iron, can slow your metabolism down and make it harder for your body to burn fat.

Solution: Eat a nutrient-dense diet rich in fruits, vegetables, and lean proteins and regularly consult with a medical practitioner to check for deficiencies.

Lacking a Regular Eating Schedule

Eating at inconsistent times can disrupt your metabolism and blood sugar levels. Skipping meals often leads to overeating later in the day.

Solution: Stick to a regular eating schedule to stabilize blood sugar and improve metabolism. Avoid skipping meals to prevent overeating later.

CHAPTER 3: BREATHING

"Breath is the bridge which connects life to consciousness, which unites your body to your thoughts."

—Thich Nhat Hanh

The importance of breathing in yoga is something that cannot be overlooked. Breathwork plays a critical role in activating the systems within the body and brings about meaningful change. With the correct type of breathwork, you can bypass the mind and enter a different state of awareness. Breathwork helps you plunge deep into your inner self, where healing takes place and love resides. Your spirit also plays a critical role here. This chapter sheds light on a few breathwork techniques you can incorporate into your meditation routine to gain a deeper sense of your inner self.

Nadi Shodhana Pranayama (Alternate Nostril Breathing)

"Nadi" is a subtle energy channel within the body that can get obstructed for many reasons, but you can unclog this channel using breathwork. The steps to do this are listed below:

1. Sit calmly with your spine in its natural curved position. Place your hands on your knees with the palms facing the ceiling.

2. Place your index and middle fingers between your eyebrows and your ring and little finger on the left nostril. Place your thumb on your right nostril. The ring finger, little finger, and thumb function as plugs that open and close the nostrils.

3. Plug your right nostril and breathe in from your left nostril. Then, plug your left nostril and breathe in from your right nostril.

4. Complete nine such rounds of breathing with your eyes closed.

Bhramari Pranayama (Bee Breath)

The sound of bee humming has great power, as it helps you feel relaxed. This exercise helps imitate bee humming to replicate the same energy within your body.

1. Sit comfortably on your chair and plug your ears with your index fingers.

2. Exhale as much air as you can and make low-pitched humming sounds.

3. Inhale and lift your fingers so your ears are opened. Keep your eyes closed throughout this exercise. You can perform bee breath up to nine times daily.

Dirga Pranayama (Three-Part Breath)

1. Place both hands on your belly such that a few fingers lie below your belly button. Notice the movement.

2. Take deep breaths and try to deepen the airflow so that your lower abdomen feels distended. Continue this phase for a sequence of five breaths.

3. Keep your right hand in its place and move your left hand toward the outer edge of your ribs. Take deep breaths, but this time, expand your belly before your ribs. Continue this motion for five consecutive calming breaths.

4. Now, slide your left hand onto your chest and take deep breaths. This time, expand your chest. These are called grounding breaths.

5. Repeat this cycle for as long as you feel comfortable.

Sama Vritti Pranayama (Equal Breathing)

This exercise can be practiced by lying on your back as well if you do not feel like doing it while sitting on a chair.

1. Find your breath. Gently breathe in and out of your lungs using diaphragmatic breathing so you breathe in and out with no movement in your chest.

2. Set your pace and breathe in and out for a specific count, such as four counts.

3. Repeat this cycle for up to 10 minutes.

Bhastrika Pranayama (Bellows Breath)

Exhale as much air as you can and inhale quickly using diaphragmatic breathing.

The gist of this exercise is to use the muscles of your diaphragm and the abdomen to force out as much air as possible and inhale the highest volume of air as quickly as possible. This exercise is very similar to equal breathing, except that you do not need to follow special sitting instructions to perform the breathing movements. You only need to be able to detect the muscles in your body that need to undergo contraction and use them to do the breathwork that is a part of this kind of yoga.

CHAPTER 4: PREPARATION

The body benefits from movement,
and the mind benefits from stillness.

—Sakyong Mipham

The succinct saying above encapsulates the state of mind that best utilizes the benefits of yoga. You need to be able to reap as much benefit as you can from your yoga practices. There is a benefit galore that comes with the right frame of mind with which you carry yourself into the world of yoga. Therefore, you need to maximize the advantage that can be reaped from your dedication to yoga. As you strap yourself tight for an adventure into your realm of yoga, do not forget to prepare the room and its surroundings, as this prepares your mind for your yoga practices.

Choosing the Right Chair, Equipment, and Clothing

The Choice of Chair

First, you need to find a sturdy chair on which to perform your yoga exercises. A sturdy chair with good and strong pedestals is an absolute necessity, and this is especially true for seniors. Yoga involves different kinds of movements wherein your body weight may shift from one edge of the chair to another. Therefore, you need to have a chair that can withstand the weight of your body as it supports it.

A wide range of chairs are available for you to choose from. Try to go to a shop that boasts having all kinds of chairs suitable for all purposes. For yoga, you need preferably a wooden chair with a slightly reclined backrest for the free movement of limbs. This way, you can lean back whenever you need a break between exercises.

Place a yoga mat beneath the chair before you start chair yoga. The mat helps the chair remain stable on the floor.

Moreover, try to push down on the chair when you buy it from the store so that you know it is stable and does not tilt along with your weight toward one side.

Clothing

Clothing is crucial when wanting to feel comfortable in general, and especially when practicing yoga. Getting into the right gear for your yoga session has immense benefits. Wear comfortable clothing that does not interfere with your movement as you transition between poses. Tight jeans and shorts tend to restrict you as you move your limbs. Try to go for loose clothing, but do not wear too baggy clothes, as they have the same restrictive effect on your movement.

Clear your surroundings of any obstacles that could interfere with the movement of your limbs. Place your chair in an open area.

Warm-Up and Cool-Down Exercises

Warming up your body enhances the benefits of yoga. Warm-up exercises primarily comprise exercises that help prepare your muscles for the strain they'll be experiencing. This helps your muscles perform yoga easily, reducing the chances of injury. While yoga comprises low-intensity movements, stretching your muscle fibers beforehand helps them move better and more comfortably.

Cooling down exercises bear similar importance and must be done after you finish your yoga session. These exercises allow you to transition into a state of rest that comprises muscle recovery. Your muscles are filled with lactic acid, especially after strenuous workouts. While yoga does not incur an oxygen debt, you must still commit to a cooling-down phase because it helps your muscles recover swiftly. These exercises consist of different techniques of meditation exercises, promoting relaxation and mental clarity alongside physical recovery.

How to Progress Week by Week

Making progress should be one of your goals in your practice. However, it is easy for us to feel stressed and pressured over workout goals because of the unrealistic beauty standards that the media feeds us. Maintaining your Chair Yoga practice as a way to get fit and get in touch with your body requires a strategy involving progressive exercises that don't put unrealistic pressure on yourself. Below are a few ways to make gentle progress in your Yoga practice.

Listening To Your Body's Signals

Pay Attention to Discomfort and Pain

Contrary to popular belief, pain and discomfort are not signs of a great workout session. Muscle soreness and pain are usually signs that you did not stretch or that you challenged yourself beyond what you were able to handle. Although it's wise to challenge yourself so that you can grow, overdoing it will actually deter your progress because you will have to pause your practice for a longer period of time to allow your muscles to heal.

Pain during your practice is also a sign that you are overworking your muscles in an unhealthy way. Pay attention to pain and discomfort, then stop to rest and check your posture and alignment to avoid injuries.

Monitor Your Breathing

Breathing is the force of life within our bodies that activates muscles and helps us shift into powerful states. Engaging in challenging movements can distract you from breathing steadily, and you may start to feel lightheaded. Always refocus on your breathing to make sure that you have enough oxygen flowing to your muscles and that you are mindful of the present moment.

Be Mindful of Fatigue and Energy Levels

During exercises, you may experience two thresholds. The first one is the mental threshold. At that stage, you will be faced with your own mental blocks and an inner critic telling you to just stop. The second threshold is your body's actual tolerance level. At that stage, you will feel fatigued, and if you push past your tolerance levels forcefully, you will get lightheaded and may injure yourself.

Pay attention to your body and your mind in order to know which threshold you are at, so you can gently support yourself either by encouraging yourself to push past mental blocks or by stopping and adding another set of movements during another Chair Yoga session.

Aspects of Yoga to Avoid

We are all likely to overstretch, so you need to check your body's limits and only twist or stretch as far as your body can bear. Weakened muscles can be subject to tears, and the pain that follows can be unbearable.

Holding a pose for too long might seem very tempting, but again, do not burden your body with something it cannot bear. Hold a pose only for as long as your body can bear the force exerted by the pose.

Seniors must avoid deep backbends, as these movements involve the back and can exert a force that is too intense to be borne in old age. Also, inversions must be avoided. These are movements wherein the head sinks below the heart's position, which can result in an undue detrimental impact on cardiovascular health.

Safe Practice

Listen to your body and learn your own limits. Do not subject your body to overexertion. Do not try to push your limits too early. Work within your limits and slowly push yourself to perform more poses or hold some poses for longer periods.

Your yoga practice must be consistent. Do not fall prey to the idea of doing more one day, as this can be very exhausting for you and result in you skipping yoga altogether the next day. Finally, remember to hydrate!

1

CHAPTER 5: EXERCISES

WARM UP

CHAIR CAT-COW STRETCH

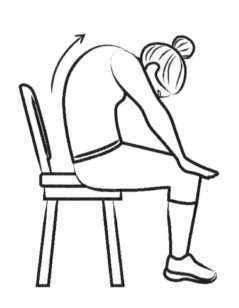 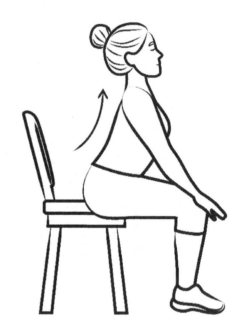

Purpose:

- This dynamic stretch promotes flexibility and mobility in the spine. It helps to relieve tension in the back and neck. The flowing movement between Cat and Cow Pose also stimulates the organs in the belly, improving digestion.

Execution:

- Sit on the edge of the chair with your feet flat on the floor.
- Place your hands on your knees or thighs.

- As you inhale, arch your back, open your chest, and lift your gaze towards the ceiling for Cow Pose.
- As you exhale, round your back, draw your belly button towards your spine, and let your head drop forward for Cat Pose.
- Continue to flow between these two poses for several breaths, moving with the rhythm of your breath.

2   NECK ROLL

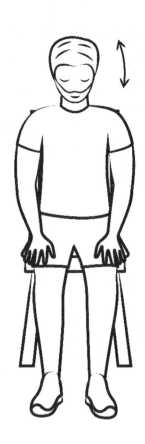
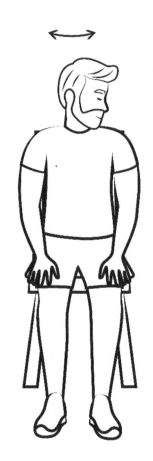

Purpose:

- Seated neck rolls not only enhance neck flexibility, but it also paves the way for improved posture, fostering overall spinal health.

Instructions

- Sit on the edge of the chair with your feet flat on the floor.
- Place your hands on your knees or thighs.
- Inhale deeply and gently lower your chin towards your chest, feeling a subtle stretch in the back of your neck.
- Slowly rotate your head to the right, aiming to bring your right ear closer to your right shoulder without straining.

- Exhale and guide your chin back to your chest in a controlled motion.
- Inhale and gently turn your head to the left, attempting to bring your left ear towards your left shoulder with ease.
- Exhale and return your chin to your chest, finalizing one full neck rotation.

3

SHOULDER SHRUGS

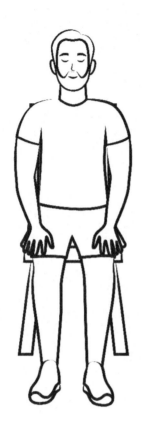 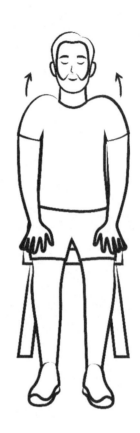

Purpose:

-   This warm-up exercise reduces tension in your traps, neck, and shoulders, preparing you fully for upcoming exercises.

Execution:

-   Sit upright with your feet shoulder-distance apart.
-   Inhale and lift your shoulders towards your ears, holding them there briefly.
-   Exhale and release the tension by slowly lowering your shoulders away from your ears.
-   Repeat the movement 5 to 10 times.

ARM CIRCLES

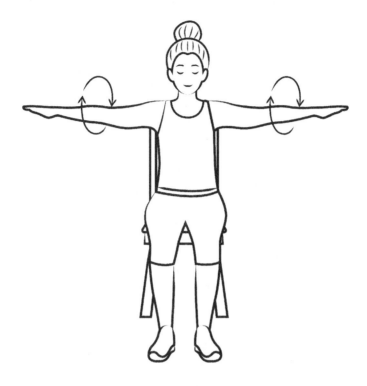

Purpose:

- Arm Circles improves flexibility and range of motion in the upper body. These circular motions also increase heart rate which improves cardiovascularity.

Execution:

- Sit on a chair with your feet shoulders distance apart.
- Slowly raise both arms out to the sides at shoulder height.
- Begin making small circular motions with both arms simultaneously.
- Bring your hands onto your knees after completing 10- 15 repetitions.
- Relax for a few breaths and then repeat the exercise, but reverse the direction of the circles this time; if you initially made clockwise circles, try counterclockwise this time.
- Make sure to control your breathing and avoid any jerky movements.

5

SEATED URDHVA HASTASANA

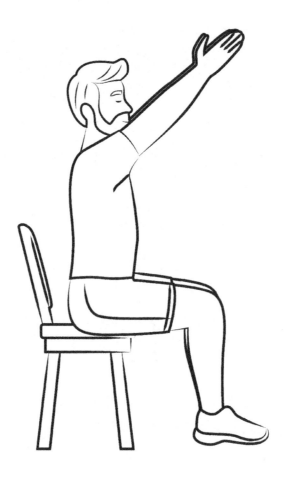

Purpose:

- The focus of this pose is to build range in your shoulder joints while using your arms as a downward driver to load and unload your upper back.

Execution:

- Sit upright on the chair. Ideally, slightly away from the backrest so that you have to use your postural muscles and core strength.
- On the inhale, raise your arms towards the ceiling while drawing your shoulder blades together and downwards.
- Imagine that you have an invisible pencil that you're trying to gently grip between your shoulder blades as you move.

- If you feel stiff and can't raise the arms all the way up, then just go as high as you can.

- Hold the arms there for a count of 20 seconds and take several controlled breaths in and out while maintaining your posture and drawing in your abs.

- Slowly lower your arms until they are at your sides. Repeat for 5 repetitions.

6

LOWER BODY

LEG PENDULUMS

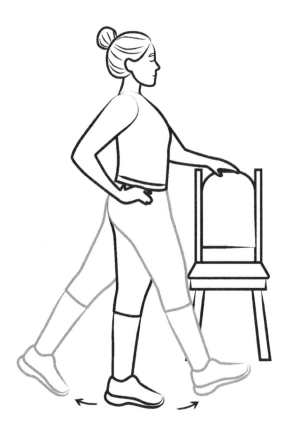

Purpose:

- This dynamic stretching exercise helps loosen up your muscles, preparing you for your chair yoga session.

Execution:

- Place one hand on a wall or hold the back of a chair for balance. Stand on one leg (keeping it straight). Swing the other leg (also straight) forward and backward 15 times.

- Switch your legs and repeat the same for the other leg.

PUSH AND STEP TO THE SIDE

7

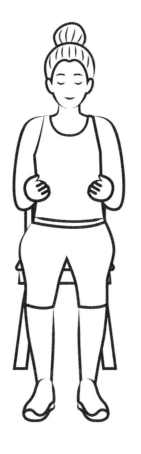 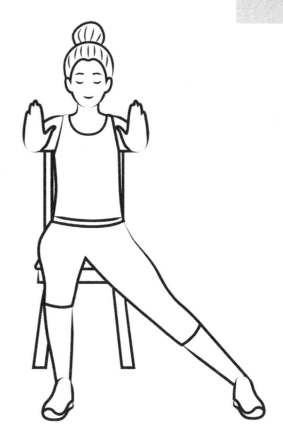

Purpose:

- This exercise targets the core, legs, and glutes, enhancing lateral stability and strength while seated.

Execution:

- Sit in the middle of the chair, closer to the edge of the seat.
- Step the right leg out and, simultaneously, push both arms out in front of you, stretch out, the palms and fingers facing up.
- Pull your arms back to your sides when the leg returns to the center.
- Emphasize the push-out and pull-back arm movement—thirty movements in total.

8

ASSISTED MARCH

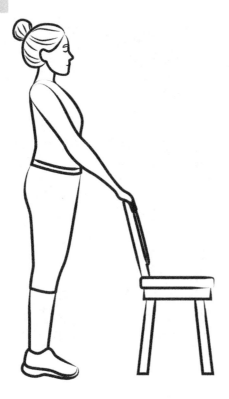 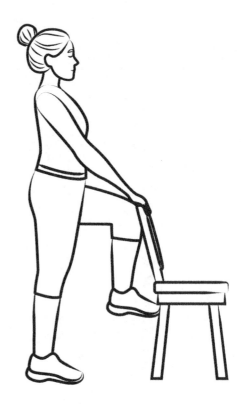

Purpose:

- This assisted march exercise elevates the heart rate, promoting cardiovascular fitness and fat burning while improving balance and coordination.

Execution:

- Stand behind the chair and put your hands on the chair's backrest for assistance.
- Lift your left knee as high as you can. Ideally with thigh parallel to the floor.
- Keep your back straight, avoiding leaning back, as you do so.
- Come back into the starting position and repeat with the other leg.
- Repeat 20-30 times in total.

CHAIR BACKWARD LUNGES

9

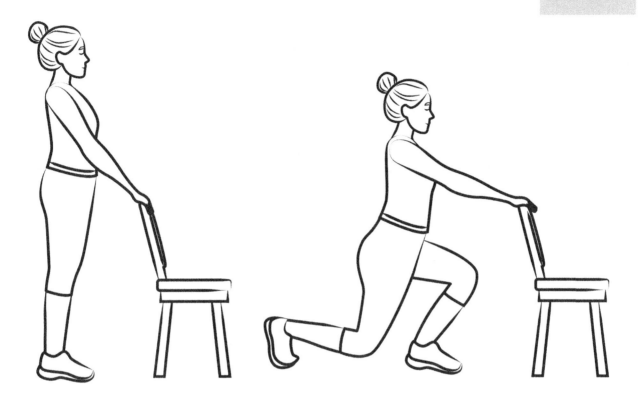

Purpose:

- This modified version of lunges strengthen the legs and glutes and promote fat burning by elevating the heart rate and engaging multiple muscle groups.

Execution:

- Stand behind the chair, holding onto the backrest for support.
- Step your right foot back into a lunge, keeping your left knee over your left ankle and your back straight.
- Lower your hips until your right knee is just above the floor, then push through your left heel to return to the starting position.
- Repeat with your left leg stepping back into a lunge.
- Continue alternating legs for 10-20 repetitions.

10 CHAIR SQUAT

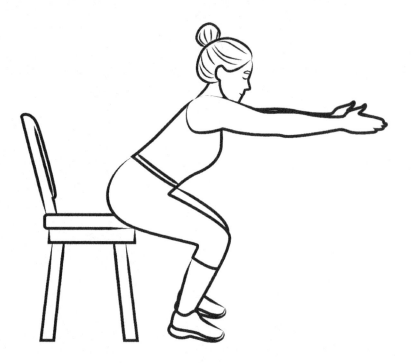

Purpose:

- Chair Squats help in strengthening the quadriceps, hamstrings, glutes, and calf muscles.

Execution:

- Begin by sitting on the edge of the chair with your feet flat on the floor, hip-width apart.
- Keep your spine tall and your shoulders relaxed.
- Inhale as you engage your core muscles and push through your heels to stand up, extending your hips and knees.
- Exhale as you slowly lower your body back down, controlling the descent and touching the chair, without sitting down. Make sure your knees are aligned with your toes, and they don't go past your toes as you lower down.
- Repeat the movement for the desired number of repetitions.

CHAIR SUPPORTED CALF RAISES

11

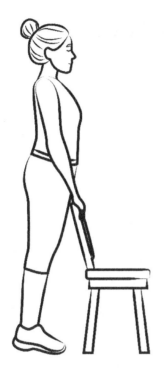 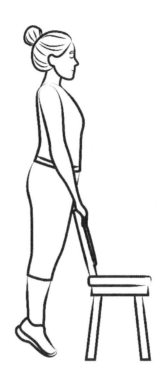

Purpose:

- This exercise strengthens the calf muscles, improves ankle stability, and can help with balance.

Execution:

- Begin standing behind your chair, resting your hands on the backrest of the chair.
- Press down into the balls of both feet to raise your heels as high as you can.
- Hold for a moment at the top, then slowly lower your heels back to the floor.
- Repeat for a set of 10-15 repetitions.

12 UPPER BODY

SEATED CACTUS POSE

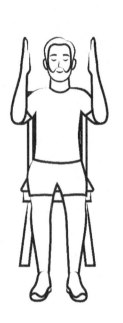 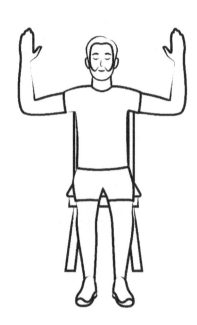

Purpose:

- This exercise helps to open up the chest and shoulders, which can become tight from hunching over. It also helps to strengthen the muscles between the shoulder blades, improving posture and stability.

Execution:

- Sit tall in your chair, feet flat on the floor. Extend your arms out to the sides at shoulder height.
- Bend your elbows to a 90-degree angle, with your palms facing forward.
- As you inhale, squeeze your shoulder blades together, opening up your chest.
- As you exhale, bring your elbows towards each other in front of you without collapsing your chest.
- Continue this opening and closing movement for several breaths.

CHAIR LIFTED HIP

13

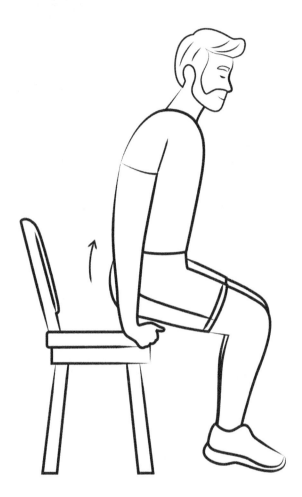

Purpose:

- This exercise strengthens the muscles of the entire upper body and core.

Execution:

- Sit with your back straight at the edge of the chair with hands at the sides of the chair for stability.
- Lift your hips from the chair by pushing with your hands on it.
- Hold that position keeping your arms straight and hips lifted up for the desired number of seconds.
- Repeat 5-10 times.

14   CHAIR PUNCHES

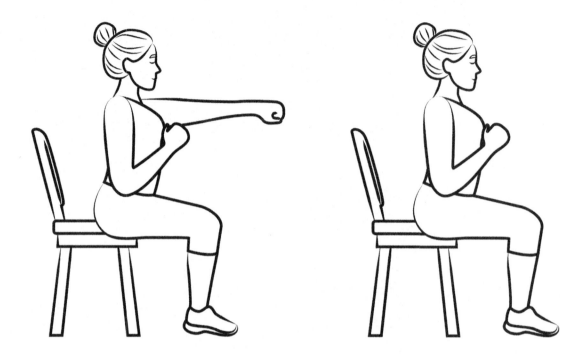

Purpose:

- This exercise promotes fat burning and cardiovascular endurance without impact on the joints.

Execution:

- Maintain an upright posture.
- Engage your core, chest, and arm muscles, ensuring a firm contraction with each swing. Position your lightly clenched fists close to your jawline.
- With control, slowly punch in front and return to the start position, then switch to the other arm.
- Alternate and repeat twenty times.

MODIFIED PUSH UP

15

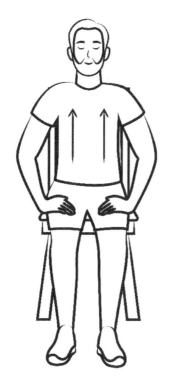
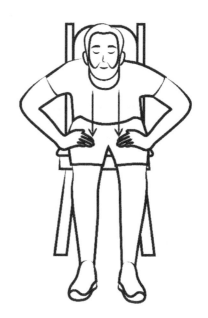

Purpose:

- This exercise offers a unique way to work on the upper body muscles.

Executions:

- Sit comfortably on a chair, positioning your legs slightly wider than hip-width apart. Ensure your feet are flat on the ground.
- Rest your hands at top of your knees, palms facing down. With a straight back, lean your chest forward towards your legs, going as low as you comfortably can.
- Engage your arms and shoulders to push yourself back to the upright starting position.
- Continue the movement for the desired number of repetitions.

16

CHAIR DIPS

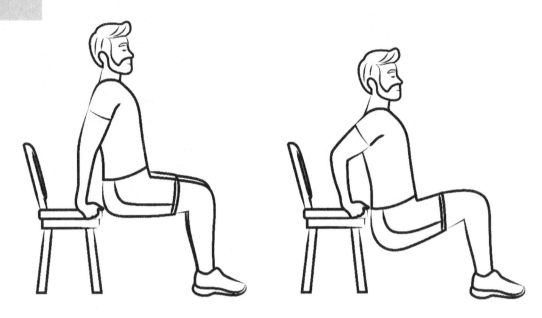

Purpose:

- Chair Dips target the triceps, shoulders, and chest muscles. They also challenge your core stability.

Execution:

- Sit on the edge of the chair and grip the front edges of the seat with your hands, knuckles facing forward.
- Walk your feet forward and slide your hips off the chair.
- Lower your body down by bending your elbows, keeping them close to your body.
- Stop when your elbows are at about a 90-degree angle or when you feel a stretch across your chest.
- Push through your hands to straighten your arms and lift your body back to the starting position.
- Repeat for the desired number of repetitions.

SHOULDER PRESS

17

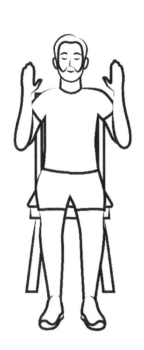 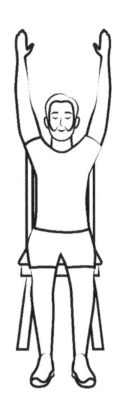

Purpose:

- This exercise also promotes better posture by engaging the muscles of the upper back and shoulders.

Execution:

- Sit on the chair with your feet flat on the floor, hip-width apart.
- Hold a pair of lightweight dumbbells or water bottles at shoulder height with your elbows bent, palms facing forward.
- Inhale to prepare, and as you exhale, press the weights overhead, extending your arms fully.
- Inhale as you slowly lower the weights back down to shoulder height.
- Repeat the movement for the desired number of repetitions.

18

ABS & CORE

SEATED SIDE STRETCH

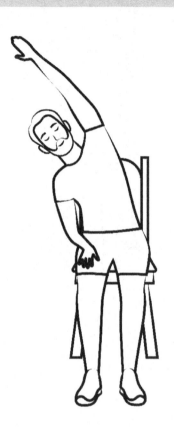 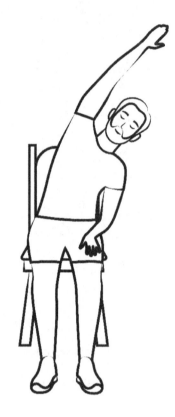

Purpose:

- This stretch opens up the side body, improving flexibility and breathing capacity. It also helps in relieving tension along the spine and in the shoulders.

Execution:

- Sit comfortably on the chair with your feet flat on the floor. Keep your spine straight and shoulders relaxed.

- Inhale deeply, and as you exhale, gently lean to the right side, sliding your right hand down the side of the chair.

- Extend your left arm overhead, reaching towards the right side, keeping your arm in line with your ear.
- Keep your chest open and your gaze towards the ceiling or straight ahead.
- Hold for a few breaths, then slowly come back to center as you inhale.
- Repeat on the other side.

19   UPWARD PLANK

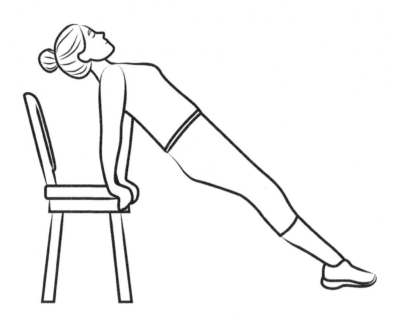

Purpose:

- This is a great pose to fix bad posture by strengthening the back and core muscles while enabling you to open your chest.

Execution:

- Sit on a chair with your feet shoulders distance apart. Place your hands directly under your shoulders on the chair with your fingers facing the front of the chair.
- Inhale and slowly extend your legs out to the front until your knees are fully locked out and your toes are pointing towards the ceiling.
- Then, push into the chair with your hands and engage your core to slightly lift yourself off of the chair until your arms are fully locked out. You should aim to get a straight, diagonal line running from your ankles to your head.
- Slightly lift your chest, point your gaze towards the ceiling, and pull your shoulder blades together.
- Hold the pose for a few deep breaths and release by bringing your hips back to the chair and then bringing your legs back to the starting position.

CHAIR PLANK

20

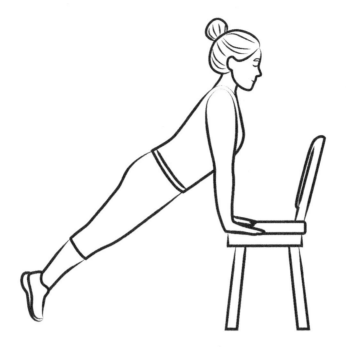

Purpose:

- Strengthens arms, shoulders, core, hips, and legs, improving endurance and stamina.

Execution:

- Stand a few steps away from a chair with your feet shoulder distance apart and place the palms of your hands on the top of the backrest of the chair.
- Pull your navel in closer to your spine to engage your core. As you breathe, step back and keep lowering yourself until your head, hips, and toes are in a straight diagonal line with your shoulders directly above your hands.
- Keep your legs engaged to prevent your hips from falling or going too high and keep your spine straight with your neck in line with it to prevent straining it.

- Hold this pose for a few breaths before releasing by walking towards the chair and lifting your torso from your back and pushing the chair with your hands until you stand tall.

- Once you get comfortable with this pose, move to start with your hands on the seat of the chair and repeat the same steps. If moving to the seat of the chair becomes too difficult, try placing your knees on the floor slowly and lift your body to build upper body strength and complete the plank pose.

LEG SHUFFLE

21

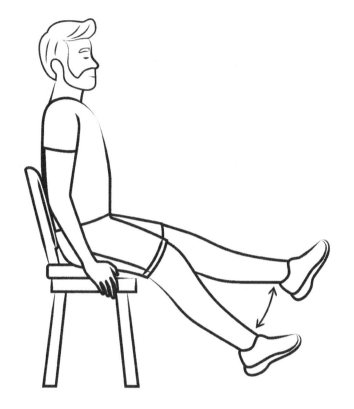

Purpose:

- Designed to strengthen the abdominal muscles and core.

Execution:

- Sit at the edge of a sturdy chair, ensuring your back is erect.
- Place your hands on either side of the chair for added stability. Gently lean your upper body backward.
- Lift both feet a few inches off the ground. Begin to shuffle your legs by moving them up and down alternately, as if marching in place.
- Maintain a steady pace and keep the movements controlled, focusing on engaging your lower abs.
- Perform the shuffle for 10-20 repetitions, rest, and repeat for 1-3 sets.

22

BRIDGE POSE

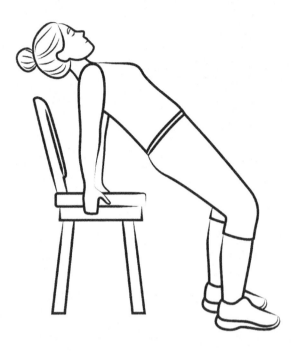

Purpose:

- Strengthens the core, glutes, and lower back muscles, which are crucial for better posture.

Execution:

- Sit on a chair with your feet shoulder-distance apart.
- Place your hands next to you on the sides of the chair for support. Next, press your feet into the ground, engage your core, and push your hands into the seat of the chair to lift your hips off the seat.
- Arch your back slightly by lifting your chest towards the ceiling and bring your shoulder blades closer to each other for stability.
- Your hands should remain directly under your shoulders, holding the weight of your upper body, and your neck should remain in line with your spine to prevent any strain on the neck.
- Hold the pose for 5 breaths before slowly lowering yourself back down to the starting position.

FLUTTER KICKS

23

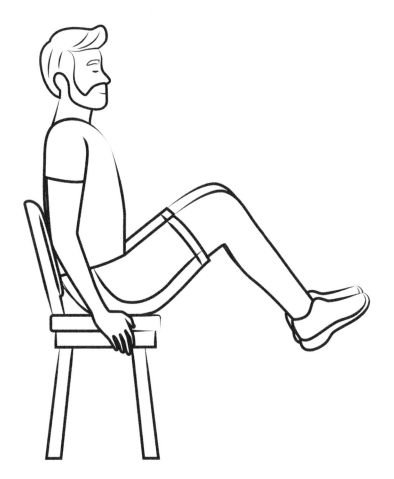

Purpose:

- This exercise strengthens the core, lower abs, and hip flexors while improving stability and balance.

Execution:

- Lean back into the chair with your spine straight.
- Fully extend your legs, hold the chair's edges, lift both legs, and flutter.
- Kick your legs up and down.
- Repeat twenty times.

24 CLASSIC YOGA POSES

TRIANGLE POSE

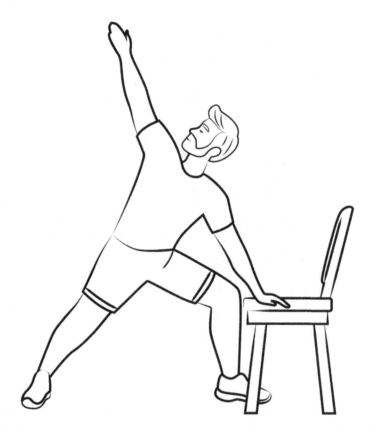

Purpose:

- Triangle pose enhances flexibility and stability in the hips and spine.

Execution:

- Stand in front of your chair facing the seat.
- Place your left foot directly in front of the chair and bring your right foot back and angled out.
- Keep a nice bend in your left leg while making sure your right leg is fully extended.

- On an exhale, drop down slightly until you have a slight bend in your left knee while keeping the right leg fully extended out to reach your left hand down to rest on the seat of the chair.

- Inhale and reach your right arm up toward the ceiling, letting your gaze follow your fingertips.

- Hold this pose for ten deep breaths.

- Repeat once more on the other side.

25

UPWARD FACING DOG

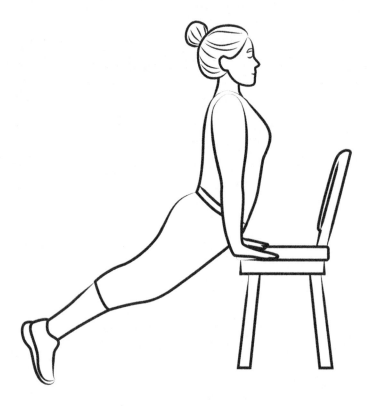

Purpose:

- This variation of upward facing dog with a chair stretches the chest, shoulders, and abdomen while relieving tension in the lower back, offering a more accessible way to improve spinal flexibility and posture.

Execution:

- Stand a couple of feet in front of your chair.
- Bend your torso down toward the chair and grab the edges of the chair's seat.
- Walk your feet back until your body is at about a 45-degree angle from the floor, with your arms straight and supporting your upper body weight.
- On an inhale, slowly bring your chest up as you arch your spine. Exhale.
- Inhale and bring your gaze up to the ceiling.
- Hold this pose for 10 deep breaths.
- Repeat this exercise once through.

STANDING HASTASAN

26

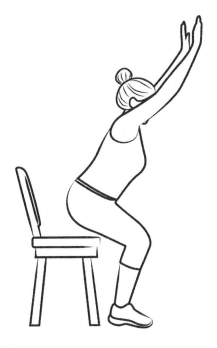

Purpose:

- Chair Pose strengthens the legs, glutes, and lower back. It also engages the core and promotes better posture.

Execution:

- Stand with your feet hip-width apart, toes pointing forward.
- Extend your arms overhead with your palms facing each other.
- As you exhale, bend your knees and lower your hips back and down as if you were going to sit in a chair. You can keep your arms raised or rest them on the back of the chair.
- Keep your chest lifted and shoulders relaxed, and avoid arching your lower back.
- Hold the pose for a few breaths, engaging your thighs and glutes.
- Inhale as you slowly stand back up to the starting position.

27 CHAIR WARRIOR POSE

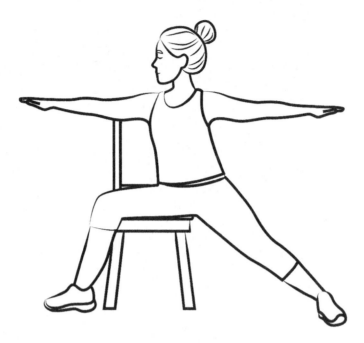

Purpose:

- Practice one of the most common yoga exercise in its modified chair version.

Execution:

- Start sitting upright on your chair, slightly over to the left-hand side of the seat.
- Turn to your right and get into a high lunge position, making sure that your right leg is supported by the chair and your left is outstretched behind.
- Turn the foot on your outstretched leg to face forward, making sure that you keep it flat on the ground. Only turn it as far as you can while remaining stable and comfortable. Take a breath in.
- Raise both arms, one in front and one behind, to shoulder height. Open your chest, lengthen your neck, and breathe out as you move.
- Focus on drawing your shoulder blades back and down.
- Hold the pose for 30 seconds while breathing normally.
- Release the pose and switch to opposite side.

SEATED SIDE LUNGE

28

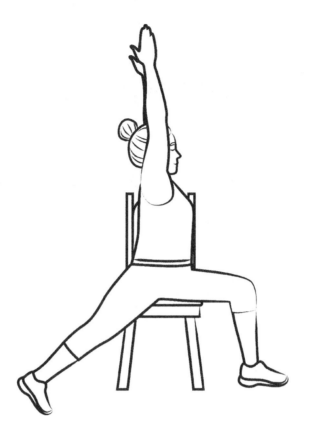

Purpose:

- This exercise is for toning and strengthening your thighs, knees, ankles, and core.

Execution:

- Sit sideways on your chair so that its backrest is next to your left arm.
- Sit toward the edge of the chair so that your left thigh is supported and your right has space to move.
- Hold onto the top of the chair's backrest with your left hand to help support you through the position. Keeping your left foot planted on the floor in front of you with its knee at 90 degrees, lengthen your right leg out behind you, perching on the ball of your right foot.
- Hold for 5 to 10 breaths before repeating on the other side.

29

CARDIO

SEATED MARCH

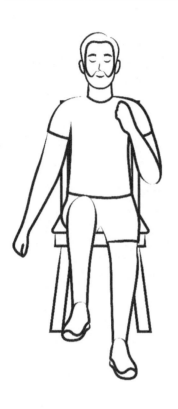 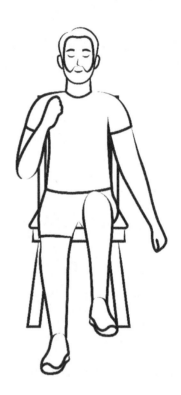

Purpose:

- Seated March is a great way to boost circulation and strengthen leg muscles. It also offers a cardiovascular workout.

Execution:

- Begin by sitting comfortably on a chair with your spine straight, feet flat on the ground, and hands resting on your thighs or by your sides.
- As you lift your right knee towards your chest, swing your left arm forward in a controlled manner, similar to a marching motion.

- Gently lower your right foot back to the ground and bring your left arm back to its starting position. Now, as you lift your left knee towards your chest, swing your right arm forward.

- Gently lower your left foot back to the ground and return your right arm to its starting position.

- Alternate between the right and left legs, mimicking a marching motion while seated, and coordinating with the opposite arm.

- Continue this marching sequence for a set number of repetitions or for a specific duration, maintaining a steady rhythm.

30

SIDE LEG RAISES

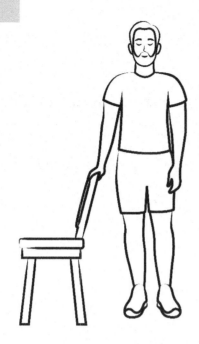 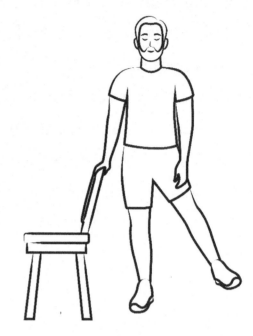

Purpose:

- Develops strong hip and upper thigh muscles, which improve overall balance and stability.

Execution:

- Stand upright with a chair on your right, keeping your shoulders relaxed and arms resting on your sides.
- Place your left hand on your waist and grab the chair with your right hand for support and balance.
- Lift your left leg out to the side by engaging your core and thigh muscles, keeping it straight.
- Hold this position for a few seconds before slowly lowering your leg back down.
- Repeat the movement for 5 repetitions before switching sides and repeating the movement with the right leg.

SEATED JUMPING JACKS

31

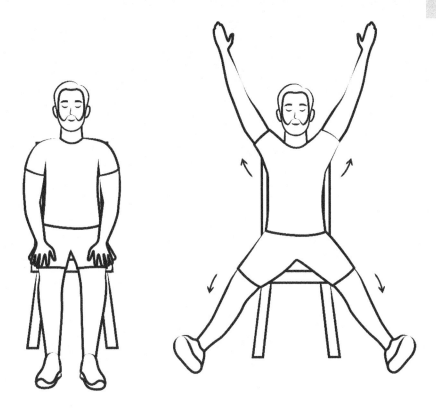

Purpose:

- Increases heart rate and breathing, which improves cardiovascular health.

Execution:

- Sit toward the front of your chair and engage your core by drawing your belly button toward your spine.
- Take a deep breath in and extend your legs out to the sides, simultaneously lifting your arms up and out to the sides.
- Your legs and arms should form a "V" shape.
- Exhale and return to the starting position by bringing your legs and arms back. Repeat for 5 to 10 repetitions, maintaining a controlled and fluid motion.

- Throughout the exercise, keep your core engaged, posture upright, and avoid slouching or leaning back into the chair.
- Gradually increase the range of motion and intensity of the movement as you become more comfortable and proficient with the exercise.

BICYCLE CRUNCHES

32

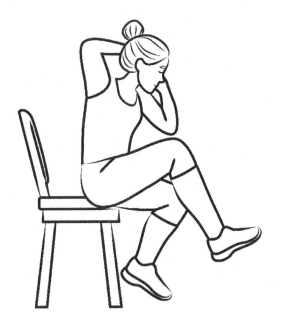 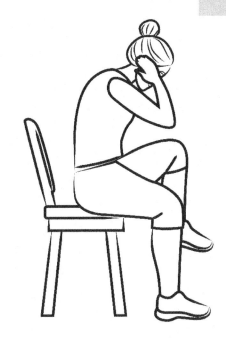

Purpose:

- Strengthens the core muscles, especially the oblique muscles, which support fat burning and weight loss.

Execution:

- Lift your right knee towards your chest while simultaneously bringing your left elbow towards it as you crunch and slightly twist your body by engaging your core muscles.
- Try to go as close as possible to touching your right knee to your left elbow and hold this position for a moment.
- Then, lower your knee back to the floor and lift your torso back up to sit straight.
- Wait for a breath and repeat on the other side (left knee to right elbow).
- Aim to alternate between the two sides for 5-10 repetitions, slowly increasing the range of your motion and speed of the movement as you get used to it.

33 MODIFIED MOUNTAIN CLIMBERS

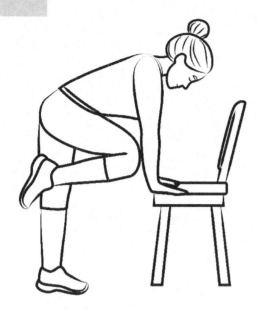 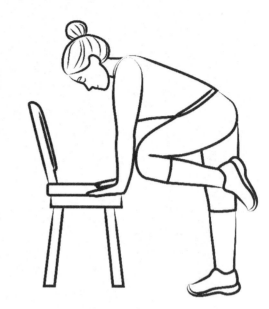

Purpose:

- Strengthens core and leg muscles, increases heart rate that helps to burn calories, and aids in weight loss.

Execution:

- Stand in front of a chair with your feet shoulder distance apart.
- Gently bend forward at your hips to lower your torso closer to the chair and place the palms of your hands on the seat of the chair.
- Next, take a deep inhale and bring your right knee close to your arms. If you can manage to touch your elbows, that's great, but do not worry if you can't, and just focus on improving your range of motion over time.
- Lower your right foot back to the ground and repeat with the other leg.
- Aim for 5 to 10 continuous alternating repetitions for 3 sets.

CHAIR JUMP ROPE

34

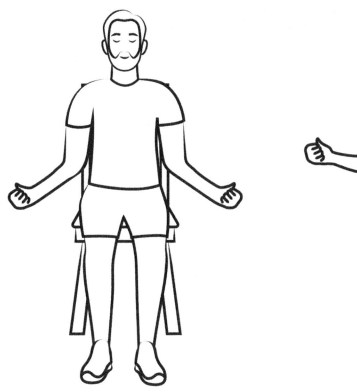 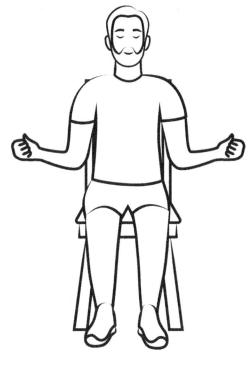

Purpose:

- Increases heart rate and breathing, which improves cardiovascular health and fat burning.

Execution:

- Sit on the chair, chest up.
- Imitate rope skipping using an imaginary rope.
- Repeat thirty times.

35 MEDITATION EXERCISES

SEATED SPHINX

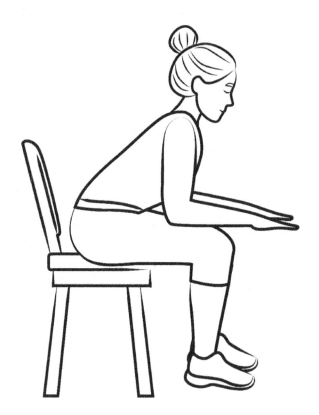

Purpose:

- Opens up the chest, which supports respiratory function by allowing the lungs to expand fully.

Execution:

- Bend forward at the hips while keeping your back straight as you slide your hands forward on your thighs.

- Simultaneously, lower your elbows to place them on your thighs. Continue bending forward until your elbows are directly below your shoulders and you form a 90-degree bend in your arms.

- Lift your chest slightly to form a slight curve in your back. Remember to keep your neck elongated and your head aligned with your spine.

- Avoid any strain or tension in your neck by keeping it relaxed. Hold the pose for 5 breaths, inhaling and exhaling steadily. Allow your breath to flow naturally and maintain a sense of relaxation throughout the pose.

- Release the pose by lifting your torso back into the starting position and then repeat for up to 3 repetitions, focusing on maintaining smooth movement.

36 | LOTUS POSE

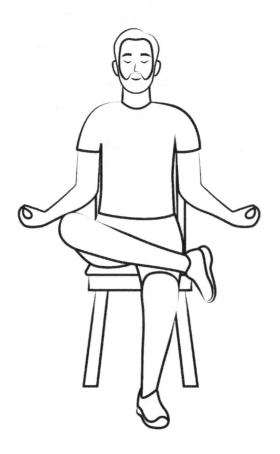

Purpose:

- Classic "calm down" yoga pose with a slight chair modification

Execution:

- Sit on a chair with your feet on the floor and your spine straight. Relax your shoulders and place your hands on your knees.
- Lift your right foot and place it on top of your left knee.
- Flex your right knee and gently press it down towards the ground, maintaining a straight spine and relaxed shoulders.
- Rest your hands on your knees, palms facing up or down.
- Take a few deep breaths and allow your body to relax in this position.
- Switch your legs halfway through the practice to balance out the stretch.

SUN BREATHS

37

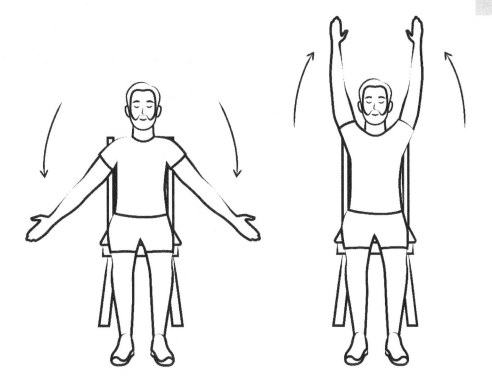

Purpose:

- The Sun Breaths pose offers a serene way to anchor oneself while deepening the connection to one's breathing.

Execution:

- Start by positioning yourself upright on a chair, ensuring your feet are firmly planted on the floor and spaced hip-width apart.

- Maintain a straight spine and let your shoulders ease into a relaxed stance.

- Initiate the exercise by drawing a deep breath in through your nostrils, allowing the inhalation to guide your movements.

- As you breathe in, lift your arms in a sweeping motion with palms facing forward. Ensure your shoulders remain at ease as you extend your arms overhead.

- When exhaling, release the breath through your nostrils slightly before you begin to lower your arms.
- Slightly rotate your palms outward as you gracefully bring your arms back down to your sides.
- Continue this pattern several times, letting each breath and movement bring you closer to a state of calm and centeredness.

PRAYER POSE

38

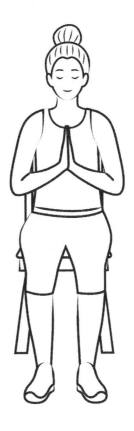

Purpose:

- Beyond fostering breath mindfulness, this pose provides a gentle stretch to the upper torso, encouraging improved posture.

Execution:

- Start by positioning yourself upright on a chair, ensuring your feet are firmly planted on the floor and spaced hip-width apart.
- Maintain a straight spine and let your shoulders ease into a relaxed stance.
- Initiate the exercise by drawing a deep breath in through your nostrils, allowing the inhalation to guide your movements.
- As you breathe in, lift your arms in a sweeping motion with palms facing forward. Ensure your shoulders remain at ease as you extend your arms overhead.

- When exhaling, release the breath through your nostrils slightly before you begin to lower your arms.
- Slightly rotate your palms outward as you gracefully bring your arms back down to your sides.
- Continue this pattern several times, letting each breath and movement bring you closer to a state of calm and centeredness.

THE GODDESS POSE

39

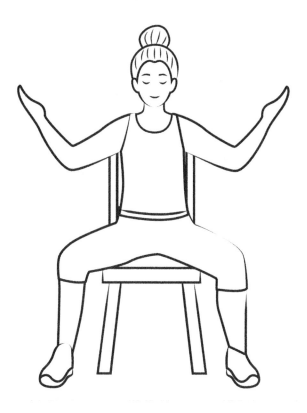

Purpose:

- A grounding pose that focuses on opening the chest and shoulders while also increasing the hip's range by stretching the adductors.

Execution:

- Spread your hips as wide as possible while splaying your feet.
- Make sure your knees are directly above your feet for proper alignment. If you have reached your maximum hip range and your knees are collapsing inward, slightly narrow your stance to correct.
- Once you are in position, move your legs outward until you feel a strong but controlled stretch. Now that your legs are in position, raise both arms laterally (out to your sides) until they are just below shoulder height, with your palms facing up.

- Bend both your arms at the elbows until they are at 90 degrees or less. Now that your arms are in position, draw your shoulder blades back and downward while lifting your chest and lengthening your neck.

- Once in the position, you will feel your chest opening outward and your spine extending.

- Now you are in a full Goddess pose, draw your abs inward to fully engage your core muscles.

- Close your eyes and breathe normally for 15 to 20 breaths before releasing.

CHAKRA

40

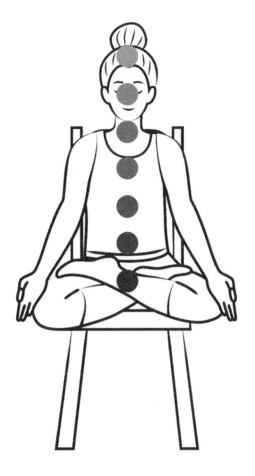

Purpose:

- Advanced meditation technique to deepen your practice and enhance spiritual growth.
- Chakras are energy centers in the body, and seven main ones are located from the base of the spine to the top of the head, representing a different aspect of our being.

Execution:

- Sit comfortably in a cross-legged position on a chair with your back straight, close your eyes, and take a few deep breaths, allowing yourself to relax.
- Begin by bringing your attention to the base of your spine, where the first chakra, the Root Chakra or Muladhara, is located. Visualize a spinning wheel

of vibrant red energy in this area, flowing freely and evenly, grounding you to the earth.

- Move your focus up to the lower abdomen, where the second chakra, Sacral Chakra or Svadhisthana, is located.

- Visualize a spinning wheel of orange energy, expanding and flowing harmoniously, enhancing your creativity and passion.

- Next to the upper abdomen, where the third chakra, the Solar Plexus Chakra or Manipura, is situated. Visualize a spinning wheel of yellow energy in this area, empowering you and strengthening your personal power and confidence.

- Then to the center of your chest, where the fourth chakra, the Heart Chakra or Anahata, is located. Visualize a spinning wheel of vibrant green energy in this area, radiating love, compassion, and harmony, both inwardly and outwardly.

- Next, to the throat, where the fifth chakra, the Throat Chakra or Vishuddha, is situated. Visualize a spinning wheel of serene blue energy in this area, clearing your communication channels and allowing you to express yourself authentically.

- Move to the space between your eyebrows, where the sixth chakra, the Third Eye Chakra or Ajna, is located. Visualize a spinning wheel of deep indigo energy and connect it with your intuition and inner wisdom as this energy center expands.

- Finally, bring your attention to the top of your head, where the seventh chakra, known as the Crown Chakra or Sahasrara, is situated.

- Visualize a spinning wheel of brilliant violet or white energy in this area, connecting you to the divine. Allow the energy to flow freely through each chakra.

- If you notice any blockage or imbalance, visualize the energy becoming clear and harmonious in those areas.
- When you are ready to conclude the meditation, take a few deep breaths and gradually bring your awareness back to your physical body.
- Gently open your eyes and take a moment to reflect on your experience.

CHAPTER 6: 28 DAY CHALLENGE

You have multiple options for progressing through this challenge, as everyone is on their own journey, starting from different levels of fitness when picking up this book. You can gradually increase the number of sets each week (in week one, complete each exercise for the day once; in week two, perform two rounds; in week three, aim for three rounds, and so on). Progressive overload is one of the most proven strategies for achieving physical transformation.

Some exercises have a range for reps or seconds. If you can push toward the higher end of the range, great—congratulations! If you manage fewer, that's perfectly fine. Remember, we're all running our own race. What's important is to stay consistent and focus on gradual improvement over time.

Day 1

Exercise	Number	Reps / Duration
Chair Cat-Cow Stretch	1	30s
Seated Side Stretch	18	5 reps
Seated cactus pose	12	15 reps
Leg Pendulums	6	15 reps
Standing Hastasan	26	30s
Seated March	29	30 reps
Seated Sphinx	35	free

Day 2

Exercise	Number	Reps / Duration
Neck Roll	2	30s
Chair Punches	14	20 reps
Bridge Pose	22	20s
Chair Squat	10	10-15 reps
Chair Warrior Pose	27	30s
Side Leg Raises	30	20-30 reps
Lotus Pose	36	free

Day 3

Exercise	Number	Reps / Duration
Shoulder Shrugs	3	20s
Flutter Kicks	23	20 reps
Modified Push Up	15	10-20 reps
Chair Supported Calf Raises	11	20 reps
Seated Side Lunge	28	30s
Seated Jumping Jacks	31	20 reps
Sun Breaths	37	free

Day 4

Exercise	Number	Reps / Duration
Arm Circles	4	15 reps
Upward Plank	19	30s
Chair Dips	16	10-20 reps
Push and Step to the Side	7	30 reps
Triangle pose	24	30s
Bicycle Crunches	32	10-15 reps
Prayer Pose	38	free

Day 5

Exercise	Number	Reps / Duration
Seated Urdhva Hastasana	5	5 reps
Chair Plank	20	20-30s
Shoulder Press	17	30 reps
Assisted March	8	30 reps
Upward Facing Dog	25	30s
Modified Mountain Climbers	33	10-15 reps
The Goddess Pose	39	free

Day 6

Exercise	Number	Reps / Duration
Chair Cat-Cow Stretch	1	30s
Leg Shuffle	21	30 reps
Chair Lifted Hip	13	10-20 reps
Chair Backward Lunges	9	20 reps
Standing Hastasan	26	30s
Chair Jump Rope	34	30 reps
Chakra	40	free

Day 7: Rest Day

Congratulations on completing your first week! Take a moment to reflect on how you feel and how the exercises have been for you. If you're feeling up for more, you can add an extra round in the next week's routine. Keep listening to your body, stay mindful, and enjoy every step of your journey!

Day 8

Exercise	Number	Reps / Duration
Neck Roll	2	30s
Seated Side Stretch	18	5 reps
Seated cactus pose	12	15 reps
Leg Pendulums	6	15 reps
Standing Hastasan	26	30s
Seated March	29	30 reps
Seated Sphinx	35	free

Day 9

Exercise	Number	Reps / Duration
Shoulder Shrugs	3	20s
Chair Punches	14	20 reps
Bridge Pose	22	20s
Chair Squat	10	10-15 reps
Chair Warrior Pose	27	30s
Side Leg Raises	30	20-30 reps
Lotus Pose	36	free

Day 10

Exercise	Number	Reps / Duration
Arm Circles	4	15 reps
Flutter Kicks	23	20 reps
Modified Push Up	15	10-20 reps
Chair Supported Calf Raises	11	20 reps
Seated Side Lunge	28	30s
Seated Jumping Jacks	31	20 reps
Sun Breaths	37	free

Day 11

Exercise	Number	Reps / Duration
Seated Urdhva Hastasana	5	5 reps
Upward Plank	19	30s
Chair Dips	16	10-20 reps
Push and Step to the Side	7	30 reps
Triangle pose	24	30s
Bicycle Crunches	32	10-15 reps
Prayer Pose	38	free

Day 12

Exercise	Number	Reps / Duration
Chair Cat-Cow Stretch	1	30s
Chair Plank	20	20-30s
Shoulder Press	17	30 reps
Assisted March	8	30 reps
Upward Facing Dog	25	30s
Modified Mountain Climbers	33	10-15 reps
The Goddess Pose	39	free

Day 13

Exercise	Number	Reps / Duration
Neck Roll	2	30s
Leg Shuffle	21	30 reps
Chair Lifted Hip	13	10-20 reps
Chair Backward Lunges	9	20 reps
Chair Warrior Pose	27	30s
Chair Jump Rope	34	30 reps
Chakra	40	free

Day 14: Rest Day

Congratulations on completing your second week! Take a moment to reflect on how you feel and how the exercises have been for you. If you're feeling up for more, you can add an extra set or round in the next week's routine. Keep listening to your body, stay mindful, and enjoy every step of your journey!

Day 15

Exercise	Number	Reps / Duration
Shoulder Shrugs	3	20s
Seated Side Stretch	18	5 reps
Seated cactus pose	12	15 reps
Leg Pendulums	6	15 reps
Standing Hastasan	26	30s
Seated March	29	30 reps
Seated Sphinx	35	free

Day 16

Exercise	Number	Reps / Duration
Arm Circles	4	15 reps
Chair Punches	14	20 reps
Bridge Pose	22	20s
Chair Squat	10	10-15 reps
Chair Warrior Pose	27	30s
Side Leg Raises	30	20-30 reps
Lotus Pose	36	free

Day 17

Exercise	Number	Reps / Duration
Seated Urdhva Hastasana	5	5 reps
Flutter Kicks	23	20 reps
Modified Push Up	15	10-20 reps
Chair Supported Calf Raises	11	20 reps
Seated Side Lunge	28	30s
Seated Jumping Jacks	31	20 reps
Sun Breaths	37	free

Day 18

Exercise	Number	Reps / Duration
Chair Cat-Cow Stretch	1	30s
Upward Plank	19	30s
Chair Dips	16	10-20 reps
Push and Step to the Side	7	30 reps
Triangle pose	24	30s
Bicycle Crunches	32	10-15 reps
Prayer Pose	38	free

Day 19

Exercise	Number	Reps / Duration
Neck Roll	2	30s
Chair Plank	20	20-30s
Shoulder Press	17	30 reps
Assisted March	8	30 reps
Upward Facing Dog	25	30s
Modified Mountain Climbers	33	10-15 reps
The Goddess Pose	39	free

Day 20

Exercise	Number	Reps / Duration
Shoulder Shrugs	3	20s
Leg Shuffle	21	30 reps
Chair Lifted Hip	13	10-20 reps
Chair Backward Lunges	9	20 reps
Seated Side Lunge	28	30s
Chair Jump Rope	34	30 reps
Chakra	40	free

Day 21: Rest Day

Congratulations on completing your third week! Take a moment to reflect on how you feel and how the exercises have been for you. If you're feeling up for more, you can add an extra set or round in the next week's routine. Keep listening to your body, stay mindful, and enjoy every step of your journey!

Day 22

Exercise	Number	Reps / Duration
Arm Circles	4	15 reps
Seated Side Stretch	18	5 reps
Seated cactus pose	12	15 reps
Leg Pendulums	6	15 reps
Standing Hastasan	26	30s
Seated March	29	30 reps
Seated Sphinx	35	free

Day 23

Exercise	Number	Reps / Duration
Seated Urdhva Hastasana	5	5 reps
Chair Punches	14	20 reps
Bridge Pose	22	20s
Chair Squat	10	10-15 reps
Chair Warrior Pose	27	30s
Side Leg Raises	30	20-30 reps
Lotus Pose	36	free

Day 24

Exercise	Number	Reps / Duration
Chair Cat-Cow Stretch	1	30s
Flutter Kicks	23	20 reps
Modified Push Up	15	10-20 reps
Chair Supported Calf Raises	11	20 reps
Seated Side Lunge	28	30s
Seated Jumping Jacks	31	20 reps
Sun Breaths	37	free

Day 25

Exercise	Number	Reps / Duration
Neck Roll	2	30s
Upward Plank	19	30s
Chair Dips	16	10-20 reps
Push and Step to the Side	7	30 reps
Triangle pose	24	30s
Bicycle Crunches	32	10-15 reps
Seated Sphinx	35	free

Day 26

Exercise	Number	Reps / Duration
Shoulder Shrugs	3	20s
Chair Plank	20	20-30s
Shoulder Press	17	30 reps
Assisted March	8	30 reps
Upward Facing Dog	25	30s
Modified Mountain Climbers	33	10-15 reps
The Goddess Pose	39	free

Day 27

Exercise	Number	Reps / Duration
Arm Circles	4	15 reps
Leg Shuffle	21	30 reps
Chair Lifted Hip	13	10-20 reps
Chair Backward Lunges	9	20 reps
Standing Hastasan	26	30s
Chair Jump Rope	34	30 reps
Chakra	40	free

Day 28 Rest Day

Congratulations on completing the 28-day Chair Yoga for Weight Loss Challenge!

CHAPTER 7:
AM/PM ROUTINES FOR WEIGHT LOSS

AM Routine 1

Welcome to your morning Chair Yoga routine! This sequence is designed to be the perfect start to your day, consisting of activation exercises that will wake up your body and prepare you for the day ahead.

You should perform this routine in 3 sets, perform each exercise for approximately 30 seconds. This structure ensures you get the most benefit from each movement, helping you feel energized and ready to take on the day.

AM ROUTINE

1. CHAIR CAT-COW STRETCH

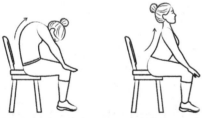

27. CHAIR WARRIOR POSE

24. TRIANGLE POSE

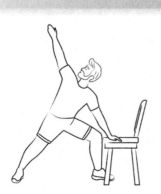

AM Routine 2

You should perform this routine in 3 sets, perform each exercise for approximately 30 seconds. This structure ensures you get the most benefit from each movement, helping you feel energized and ready to take on the day.

AM ROUTINE

5. SEATED URDHVA HASTASANA

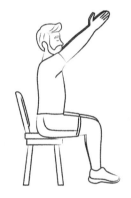

27. CHAIR WARRIOR POSE

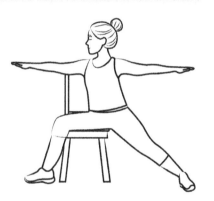

22. BRIDGE POSE

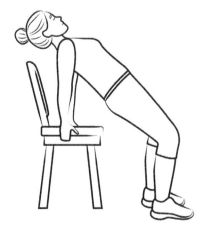

AM Routine 3

You should perform this routine in 3 sets, perform each exercise for approximately 30 seconds. This structure ensures you get the most benefit from each movement, helping you feel energized and ready to take on the day.

AM ROUTINE

7. PUSH AND STEP TO THE SIDE

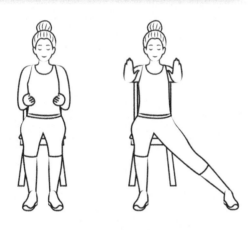

26. STANDING HASTASAN

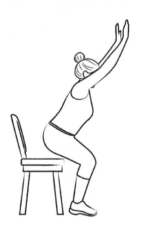

25. UPWARD FACING DOG

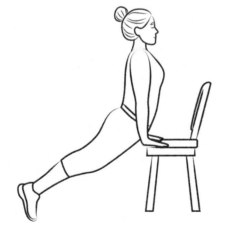

PM Routine 1

Welcome to your evening Chair Yoga routine! This sequence is centered around meditative exercises that will help you unwind and relax after a long day, preparing your mind and body for a restful night's sleep.

You should perform this routine in 3 sets, perform each exercise for approximately 30 seconds. This structure ensures you get the most benefit from each movement, helping you to calm your mind and soothe your body before bedtime.

Feel free to stay in the final pose of the last set for as long as you like, allowing the stillness to deepen your meditation. Let go of all thoughts and simply be. After the calming sequence you've just completed, you are now fully relaxed and ready for a restful, healthy sleep.

PM ROUTINE

12. SEATED CACTUS POSE

38. PRAYER POSE

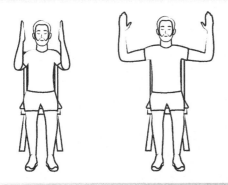

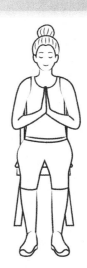

35. SEATED SPHINX

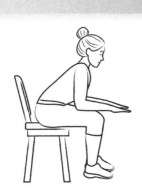

PM Routine 2

You should perform this routine in 3 sets, perform each exercise for approximately 30 seconds. This structure ensures you get the most benefit from each movement, helping you to calm your mind and soothe your body before bedtime.

Feel free to stay in the final pose of the last set for as long as you like, allowing the stillness to deepen your meditation. Let go of all thoughts and simply be. After the calming sequence you've just completed, you are now fully relaxed and ready for a restful, healthy sleep.

PM ROUTINE

2. NECK ROLL

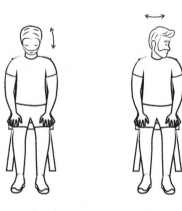

40. CHAKRA

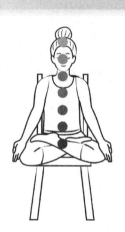

39. THE GODDESS POSE

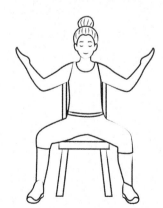

PM Routine 3

You should perform this routine in 3 sets, perform each exercise for approximately 30 seconds. This structure ensures you get the most benefit from each movement, helping you to calm your mind and soothe your body before bedtime.

Feel free to stay in the final pose of the last set for as long as you like, allowing the stillness to deepen your meditation. Let go of all thoughts and simply be. After the calming sequence you've just completed, you are now fully relaxed and ready for a restful, healthy sleep.

PM ROUTINE

37. SUN BREATHS

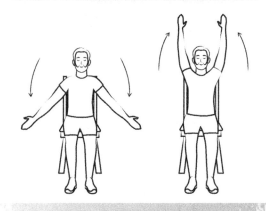

36. LOTUS POSE

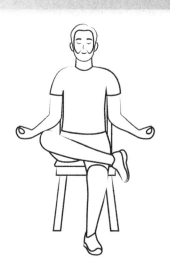

35. SEATED SPHINX

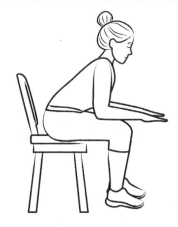

BONUS CHAPTER 1: MEDITATION

In meditation, the mind is clear, relaxed, and inwardly focused. When you meditate, you are fully awake and alert, but your mind is not focused on the external world or on the events taking place around you.

—Lama Surya Das

The power of the mind over the body is a force to be reckoned with, and meditation allows you to tap into that power. Meditative practices have a resounding impact on the way your inner self manifests. Finding that sense of peace within yourself enables you to explore the deeper pits within your shadow self that you try to keep buried, and in doing so, you become a stronger and more resilient version of yourself.

Cultivating awareness of the self is imperative to reap the benefits of yoga, and meditation and yoga go hand in hand to allow you to reach that degree of self-awareness. Knowing the elements that define you can help you work on your growth and become a superior version of your former self.

Augmenting the Mind–Body Connection

Yoga and meditation have a considerable overlap in cultivating a sense of inner peace. While yoga focuses on physical movements and dedication to the postures (asana), meditation focuses on the mental realm. Meditation helps you clear your mind of everyday clutter. It helps to sow the seeds of inner peace and the ability to find yourself and conquer it. When you conquer your weaknesses and everything that holds you back from becoming the person you want to be, the path ahead of you illuminates and leads you to your destination. You become more satisfied with yourself, and the goals you once set for yourself become more tangible.

A sense of inner stillness is necessary to concentrate on any task. This is why the significance of meditation cannot be weighed lightly on any scale. If you meditate daily, your focus improves and the turnaround time of any task allocated to you is shortened.

It is preferable to meditate before you perform yoga. This is because it clears up your mind and helps you focus more intently on the postures of yoga, also known as asanas. Moreover, it can help you feel energetic. Mindfulness is a highly sought-after attribute for your personality and can be enhanced through meditation and yoga. Practicing both together daily produces a synergistic effect on an unimaginable scale. The connection between your mind and body grows and you find deeper contentment in your daily activities.

Together, meditation and yoga can help reduce stress significantly. Meditation calms the nerve centers and helps lower cortisol levels in the bloodstream, which helps you feel more at peace with yourself. When you find a sense of inner peace, you tend to focus more easily on whatever you have to do and find joy in everything life has to offer. Additionally, you develop a positive outlook that helps you find an upside to every facet of life, even the calamities that befall you.

Emotional regulation is another byproduct of meditation. As a result of committing to a life composed of meditation, you tend to process the gamut of emotional situations in a way that contributes to your emotional intelligence. Expressing the right emotions in the face of life-changing events makes your social image more robust. Furthermore, it allows you to be aware of your hidden emotions that might interfere with daily activities. Acknowledging these emotions and regulating them becomes possible through meditation as you tap into the latent potential of your inner self. The power of your inner self is very potent, and meditation helps make it even more so to help you become strong enough to tackle anything life throws at you. This is why meditation is highly recommended for those of us who ardently commit to yoga practices.

How to Start

Find a quiet place and set a time limit for yourself. Sit cross-legged on the floor and focus on your body and breath. If your mind wanders, bring your attention back to your breath. If your mind wanders recursively, do not judge yourself, just return your focus to your breaths. Finally, open your eyes and listen to your surroundings. Notice how your body feels after this phase.

Try to commit to this practice at the same time every day and do it consistently. Moreover, work on increasing the time you spend meditating. If you start by meditating for 15 minutes every day, try increasing this time by 5 minutes every week.

BONUS CHAPTER 2: SLEEP

Yoga is the perfect opportunity to be curious about who you are. Sleep allows the inner exploration to deepen, rejuvenating the body and mind.

—Jason Crandell

Recent scientific discoveries have revealed the importance of sleep. Scientists argue that the body undergoes repair when asleep, allowing the cells to dispose of worn-out protoplasmic structures and make new ones. The brain processes and stores valuable experiences and important information learned throughout the day. More profound sleep leads to better lives wherein you enjoy every moment.

The Circadian Rhythm and Sleep Pattern

The circadian rhythm (biological clock) of your body makes you fall asleep at specific times, and you need to adhere to it to allow yourself some good sleep. Go to bed early and get up early in the morning to fully reap the benefits of yoga, as you cannot do so if your body is tired. You need to adjust your sleep pattern in a way that aligns with your natural circadian rhythm, which is the same for all of us and is about getting up to seven to eight hours of sleep a day. Try to go to bed and get up at the same time every day to regulate your biological clock.

Exposure to the Sun

Expose yourself to the sun as soon as you wake up so that the hormone serotonin surges through your bloodstream. Serotonin helps you feel energetic and full of vigor, which allows you to commit to your daily activities with greater energy. Serotonin levels in the body are subject to the regulation of the circadian rhythm.

If you have a massive disruption in your sleep pattern, you are likely to have your serotonin levels undergo fluctuations. This predisposes you to mood swings and results in a lack of energy to commit to everyday tasks, which is why adjusting your sleep routine is important.

Caffeine Intake

Caffeine intake can cause a serious disruption in the regulation of sleep patterns. Avoid consuming caffeine close to your bedtime or in the evenings. If you really need to drink coffee or tea, do it early in the day. Consuming any caffeinated drinks later in the day makes you subject to sleep disturbances. Some people might not be able to sleep at all after consuming coffee in the evening.

Shutting Out Sources of Disruption

Your bedroom is supposed to be a place where you can sleep without any disturbances. Therefore, it is better not to have a television or other sources of entertainment in this space. It is good if you happen to be someone who can exercise self-control, but many people cannot do this and succumb to the idea of watching a bit of their favorite program just when the clock ticks toward the time of hitting the hay. This habit can wreak havoc on your bedtime routine. Also, instead of watching TV, try to commit to a habit of bedtime rituals that predispose you to a more profound state of sleep. This can include having a warm bath before you go to bed. Warm showers calm the nerves and make you fall asleep.

The Importance of Bedtime Rituals

Disconnect from the internet and any devices around you. We do not realize the detrimental impact of social media and the internet on our sense of tranquility and productivity. Try disconnecting yourself from the web before you go to bed. Also, you can use some essential oils in your bedroom to help you fall asleep. Lavender oil can calm the nerves and help induce sleep. Commit to these habits to maximize the benefits of yoga. It is a good habit to get into reading books and novels before going to bed.

Ventilation in Your Bedroom

The flow of air into and out of your room has monumental importance. If hot air builds up in your space, especially during the summer season, you will eventually resort to using air conditioning more often, but you can cut down on that if you find time to let air pass through your room every day. This helps to cool down your room and prevent odors from developing due to inadequate ventilation.

Snacking at Bedtime

Always try to have your meals two or three hours before bed. Going to bed with a belly filled with food yet to be digested can lead to discomfort and reduced sleep quality.

The Integrity of Your Sleep Temple

Consider your bedroom your sleep temple. You'll need to remove television sets and any digital devices that keep you hooked to the internet. Also, when using screens, try to put on blue light filtering glasses, as blue light from screens can be a source of agitation. It is best to put your cellphone into airplane mode, so you are not disturbed by the EMF radiation during the night.

Spending Time in Nature

Devote some time to interact with nature, as this helps to regulate your biochemical processes. Go to the beach or spend time in a garden. This can really help soothe your senses and nerves. Even grounding yourself by walking barefoot can help you feel better. In fact, when your connection to the Earth is restored through grounding, electrons flood throughout your body, reducing inflammation and oxidative stress while also reinforcing your body's defense mechanisms. Electron transfers are the basis of virtually all antioxidant and anti-inflammatory activity. This is why spending time in nature can feel truly meditative and relaxing.

3 SECRET BONUSES

To get your ALL 3 SECRET BONUSES FOR FREE, just **scan the QR code above or enter this link**: https://bit.ly/CYWL-bonuses into your search browser.

Curious about the 3 BONUSES?

- ✓ **Printable 28-Day Challenge Yoga Chart with Images:** The chart becomes truly helpful once you've mastered the exercises using the book's detailed instructions, allowing you to simply glance at the images and follow the routine without flipping through pages. All exercises for the entire challenge are displayed on a single, easy-to-follow page!

- ✓ **How to Create a Habit:** Learn the proven strategies to build lasting habits that will transform your health and wellness journey.

- ✓ **Simple Biohacks to Live Longer:** Discover easy, science-backed tips to enhance your vitality and longevity effortlessly.

And as a token of my appreciation, I'm also gifting you all my future books for free because I genuinely care about your journey.

Prepare to take your fitness to the next level!

Yours truly, Alex.

CONCLUSION

Committing to a yoga routine without preparation is like setting out on a journey without a plan. While many people today focus on improving their health and daily habits, turning those intentions into lasting results requires dedication and persistence. It's not just about wanting a healthier lifestyle—it's about knowing how to make these practices a natural part of your daily life.

Yoga demands consistency and commitment to reach the goals you set for yourself. The real key is building a habit and sticking with it, even when challenges arise. By showing up each day and trusting the process, you'll see the progress unfold over time.

Thank you for allowing me to be a part of your fitness journey. Remember, the only limits are the ones you place on yourself—stay committed, and keep pushing forward!

HELP ME SPREAD THE WORD

I hope you've found valuable insights in this book and have been able to put the challenges into action. If this book has been helpful on your journey, I would truly appreciate it if you could leave a review on Amazon. I'd love to hear about the transformations you've experienced by applying the content in your daily life.

Your feedback inspires me to keep creating material that supports you in reaching your goals and improving your health. It has been a pleasure to be a part of your fitness journey. Keep pushing forward, and know that I'm cheering for your continued success!

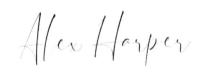

REFERENCES

Bilski, R. (2019, February 25). *Dirgha pranayama: An introduction to 3 part breathing.* Yogapedia.com. https://www.yogapedia.com/dirgha-pranayama-an-introduction-to-three-part-breath/2/11311

Nadi shodhan pranayama | How to do & benefits of nadi shodhan. (2023, June 18). Artofliving.org. https://www.artofliving.org/in-en/yoga/pranayama/nadi-shodhan-alternate-nostril-breathing

Williams, S. (2019, April 24). *What Is chair yoga? Benefits, poses & more.* Yoga Practice. https://yogapractice.com/yoga/what-is-chair-yoga/

Abdulrhman, M., El-Hefnawy, M., Hussein, R., & El-Goud, A. A. (2013). The glycemic and peak incremental indices of honey, sucrose and glucose in patients with type 1 diabetes mellitus: effects on C-peptide level-a pilot study. *Acta Diabetologica, 48*(2), 89-94. https://doi.org/10.1007/s00592-009-0167-7

Bogdanov, S., Jurendic, T., Sieber, R., & Gallmann, P. (2008). Honey for nutrition and health: a review. *Journal of the American College of Nutrition, 27*(6), 677-689. https://doi.org/10.1080/07315724.2008.10719745

Calder, P. C. (2013). Omega-3 polyunsaturated fatty acids and inflammatory processes: Nutrition or pharmacology? *British Journal of Clinical Pharmacology, 75*(3), 645–662. https://doi.org/10.1111/j.1365-2125.2012.04374.x

Fernandes, G., Velangi, A., & Wolever, T. M. (2005). Glycemic index of potatoes commonly consumed in North America. *Journal of the American Dietetic Association, 105*(4), 557-562. https://doi.org/10.1016/j.jada.2005.01.003

Fernández, M., Hudson, J. A., Korpela, R., & de los Reyes-Gavilán, C. G. (2015). Impact on human health of microorganisms present in fermented dairy products: An overview. *BioMed Research International,* 2015, 412714. https://doi.org/10.1155/2015/412714

Frisard, M. I., Broussard, A., Davies, S. S., Roberts, L. J., Rood, J., de Jonge, L., Fang, X., Jazwinski, S. M., Deutsch, W. A., & Ravussin, E. (2007). Aging, resting metabolic rate, and oxidative damage: results from the Louisiana healthy aging study. *The Journals of Gerontology Series A: Biological Sciences and Medical Sciences, 62*(7), 752-759. https://doi.org/10.1093/gerona/62.7.752

Gonzalez, J. T., Veasey, R. C., Rumbold, P. L., & Stevenson, E. J. (2013). Breakfast and exercise contingently affect postprandial metabolism and energy balance in physically active males. *British Journal of Nutrition, 110*(4), 721-732. https://doi.org/10.1017/S0007114512005582

Hall, K. D., Heymsfield, S. B., Kemnitz, J. W., Klein, S., Schoeller, D. A., & Speakman, J. R. (2012). Energy balance and its components: Implications for body weight regulation. *The American Journal of Clinical Nutrition, 95*(4), 989-994. https://doi.org/10.3945/ajcn.112.036350

Hijikata, Y., & Yamada, S. (2011). Walking just after a meal seems to be more effective for weight loss than waiting for one hour to walk after a meal. *International Journal of General Medicine, 4*, 447-450. https://doi.org/10.2147/IJGM.S18837

Howarth, N. C., Saltzman, E., & Roberts, S. B. (2001). Dietary fiber and weight regulation. *Nutrition Reviews, 59*(5), 129-139. https://doi.org/10.1111/j.1753-4887.2001.tb07001.x

Keenan, M. J., Zhou, J., Hegsted, M., Pelkman, C., Durham, H. A., Coulon, D. B., & Martin, R. J. (2015). Role of resistant starch in improving gut health, adiposity, and insulin resistance. *Advances in Nutrition, 6*(2), 198-205. https://doi.org/10.3945/an.114.007419

Kinsey, A. W., & Ormsbee, M. J. (2015). The health impact of nighttime eating: old and new perspectives. *Nutrients, 7*(4), 2648-2662. https://doi.org/10.3390/nu7042648

Leidy, H. J., Ortinau, L. C., Douglas, S. M., & Hoertel, H. A. (2013). Beneficial effects of a higher-protein breakfast on appetite, hunger, and subsequent eating behavior. *The American Journal of Clinical Nutrition, 97*(4), 677-688. https://doi.org/10.3945/ajcn.112.053132

Ludwig, D. S. (2002). The glycemic index: physiological mechanisms relating to obesity, diabetes, and cardiovascular disease. *JAMA, 287*(18), 2414-2423. https://doi.org/10.1001/jama.287.18.2414

Rautiainen, S., Wang, L., Lee, I. M., Manson, J. E., Buring, J. E., & Sesso, H. D. (2016). Dairy consumption in association with weight change and risk of becoming overweight or obese in middle-aged and older women: a prospective cohort study. *The American Journal of Clinical Nutrition, 103*(4), 979-988. https://doi.org/10.3945/ajcn.115.118406

Scazzina, F., Del Rio, D., Pellegrini, N., & Brighenti, F. (2009). Sourdough bread: Starch digestibility and postprandial glycemic response. *Journal of Cereal Science, 49*(3), 419-421. https://doi.org/10.1016/j.jcs.2008.12.008

Westerterp, K. R. (2004). Diet-induced thermogenesis. *Nutrition & Metabolism, 1*(1), 5. https://doi.org/10.1186/1743-7075-1-5

Printed in Great Britain
by Amazon

60603545R00065